Dandruff Decoded

Navigating Causes, Treatments, and Prevention

Dr Mukesh Aggarwal

CONTENTS

PREFACE

Dandruff, an age-old concern, has perplexed and troubled many individuals across generations. Despite its prevalence, the nuances of this condition often remain enigmatic, leading to misconceptions and frustration.

In this comprehensive guide, "Dandruff Decoded," Dr. Mukesh Aggarwal delves deep into the multifaceted realm of dandruff. From its fundamental understanding to the intricate science behind its occurrence, this book aims to demystify the complexities surrounding dandruff.

Through an exploration of its causes, types, symptoms, and diagnosis, this book endeavors to equip readers with the knowledge needed to identify and comprehend this common scalp condition. Dr. Aggarwal navigates the landscape of available treatments, from home remedies to professional therapies, offering insights into managing and preventing dandruff effectively.

Furthermore, this book does not merely confine itself to the physical manifestations of dandruff. It delves into the psychological impact of this condition, explores its intersection with other skin conditions, and provides considerations for special cases, such as dandruff in children.

Lastly, **"Dandruff Decoded"** peeks into the future, offering a glimpse into ongoing research, potential breakthroughs, and the innovative treatments that might redefine how we perceive and treat dandruff.

May this book serve as a guiding light, empowering readers with knowledge and strategies to combat dandruff and embrace a healthier scalp with confidence.

With warm regards
Dr Mukesh Aggarwal

UNDERSTANDING DANDRUFF

WHAT IS DANDRUFF?

Dandruff is a prevalent scalp condition that manifests as the shedding of dead skin cells from the scalp. It presents itself as white, flaky particles that can be noticeable on hair, shoulders, or clothing. While it's a harmless condition, it can be embarrassing and sometimes uncomfortable.

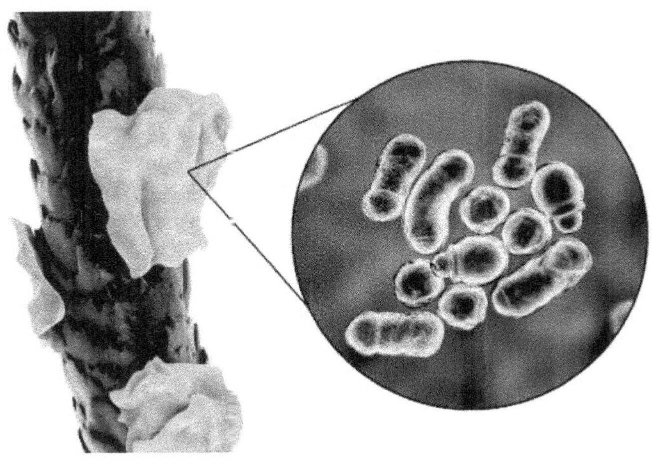

The symptoms of dandruff include white or yellow flakes on the scalp, itching, and a feeling of tightness in the scalp. It's essential to differentiate between dandruff and other conditions like dry scalp or product residue, as the treatment approach can differ.

Managing dandruff typically involves using anti-dandruff shampoos that contain active ingredients like zinc pyrithione, selenium sulfide, ketoconazole, and herbal extract coal tar. These ingredients help reduce the growth of the fungus and slow down the shedding of skin cells. Regular and proper hair care, including gentle cleansing and avoiding harsh products can also help manage dandruff.

CAUSES AND TRIGGERS OF DANDRUFF

Dandruff, a bothersome scalp condition characterized by flaking skin, can be triggered by various factors. Understanding these causes and triggers is crucial in managing and preventing its occurrence.

Dry Skin: One of the primary reasons for dandruff is dry skin. When the scalp becomes excessively dry, it leads to flaking and shedding of dead skin cells. This can be exacerbated by environmental factors like cold weather or using harsh hair care products.

Seborrheic Dermatitis: This is a chronic skin condition that causes red, itchy, and flaky skin, mainly on the scalp but also on other oily areas like the face and upper chest. Seborrheic dermatitis can contribute significantly to dandruff formation.

Malassezia: A naturally occurring fungus found on the scalp, Malassezia, can contribute to dandruff. An overgrowth of this fungus can irritate the scalp, leading to an increased turnover of skin cells and the characteristic flaking.

Sensitive Skin and Allergic Reactions: Some individuals have sensitive skin that reacts adversely to certain hair care products or ingredients. Allergic reactions or sensitivities to shampoos, hair dyes, or other hair care products can cause scalp irritation, resulting in dandruff.

Poor Hygiene: Not cleaning the scalp regularly or not washing the hair enough can lead to a buildup of oil, dead skin cells, and product residue. This buildup can create an environment conducive to dandruff formation.

Diet and Stress: While the direct correlation is not entirely clear, some studies suggest that diet and stress levels can impact dandruff. Poor diet or high stress might compromise the immune system, potentially exacerbating scalp conditions.

Hormonal Changes: Fluctuations in hormones, particularly during puberty, pregnancy, or due to certain medical conditions, can influence the production of oil in the skin and consequently trigger dandruff.

Understanding these causes and triggers of dandruff is crucial in adopting an effective treatment and prevention strategy. Using specialized anti-dandruff shampoos, maintaining good scalp hygiene, managing stress levels, and being mindful of product choices can help in managing and preventing the recurrence of dandruff. Consulting a dermatologist for severe or persistent cases is advisable to determine the most suitable treatment plan.

COMMON MISCONCEPTIONS ABOUT DANDRUFF

Dandruff, a prevalent scalp condition, is often surrounded by various misconceptions that can lead to misunderstanding and improper management of the condition. Addressing these misconceptions is essential in fostering a better understanding of dandruff.

Dandruff is Caused by Poor Hygiene: Contrary to popular belief, dandruff is not solely caused by poor hygiene. While inadequate scalp hygiene can contribute to dandruff, it's not the only factor. Factors like dry skin, fungal overgrowth, or skin conditions play significant roles in its development.

Dandruff is Contagious: Dandruff is not contagious. It's a common scalp condition caused by various factors like dry skin, fungal activity, or sensitivity to hair products. It cannot be transmitted from person to person through direct contact or sharing personal items.

Dandruff Only Affects the Scalp: While dandruff primarily manifests on the scalp as flaking skin, it can sometimes impact other areas with high oil secretion, like the eyebrows, ears, and sides of the nose. It's not confined solely to the scalp.

Dandruff is Always Caused by Dry Skin: While dry skin is a common cause of dandruff, it's not the only culprit. Other factors, including excessive oil production, sensitivity to hair products, fungal infections like Malassezia, or skin conditions such as seborrheic dermatitis, can also lead to dandruff.

Using More Shampoo Eliminates Dandruff: Overwashing or using excessive shampoo doesn't necessarily cure dandruff. In some cases, harsh shampoos can irritate the scalp, exacerbating the condition. Using specialized anti-dandruff shampoos in moderation and as directed is more effective.

Dandruff is Untreatable: While dandruff can be persistent, it's treatable and manageable. Anti-dandruff shampoos containing active ingredients like zinc pyrithione, selenium sulfide, ketoconazole, or coal tar can effectively control and reduce dandruff when used consistently.

Scratching Removes Dandruff: Scratching the scalp to remove dandruff can worsen the condition. It may lead to scalp irritation and potentially cause small wounds, making the scalp more susceptible to infections.

Understanding the actual causes and appropriate management strategies for dandruff is crucial in dispelling these misconceptions. Seeking advice from dermatologists or healthcare professionals can provide accurate information and personalized treatment plans for effectively managing dandruff.

Chapter 2

THE SCIENCE BEHIND DANDRUFF

Dandruff is often caused by an overgrowth of a yeast-like fungus called Malassezia, which feeds on the natural oils produced by your scalp. This overgrowth can lead to skin cells shedding more quickly, resulting in the characteristic flakes. Other factors like dry skin, sensitivity to hair products, or certain skin conditions can also contribute to dandruff.

SCALP ANATOMY AND FUNCTIONS

The scalp is a crucial part of the body, providing essential functions and housing intricate anatomy. Comprised of layers, structures, and functions, it plays a pivotal role in protection, sensation, and hair growth.

ANATOMY:

Skin Layers: The scalp consists of five layers of skin: the epidermis, dermis, hypodermis, galea aponeurotica, and periosteum. The epidermis is the outermost layer, providing a protective barrier, while the dermis contains hair follicles, sebaceous glands, and blood vessels. The hypodermis houses fat cells and connects the scalp to the skull.

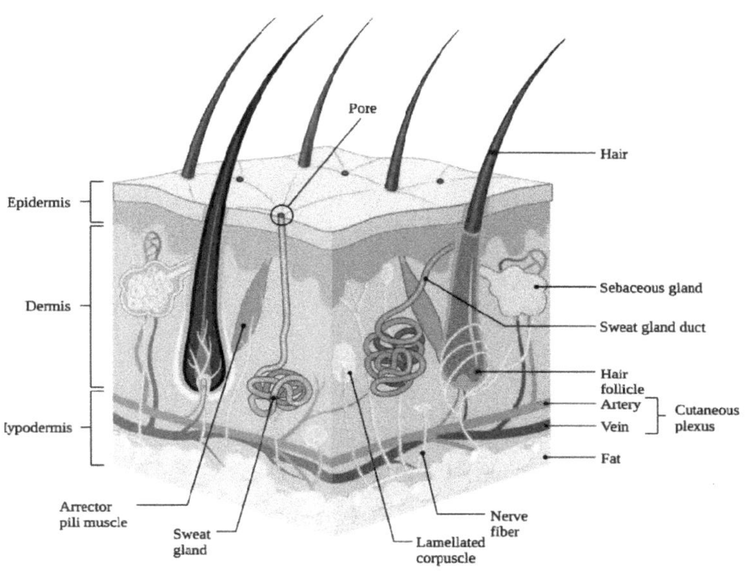

Hair Follicles: These are complex structures within the dermis responsible for hair growth. Each follicle includes the hair bulb, papilla, and sebaceous gland. Hair grows from the bulb, and sebaceous glands produce sebum, an oily substance that moisturizes and protects the hair.

FUNCTIONS:

Protection: The scalp shields the skull from external trauma, UV radiation, and temperature fluctuations. Hair also provides insulation and helps maintain body heat.

Sensation: Nerves in the scalp allow for sensory perception, including touch, pressure, and temperature.

These sensations aid in detecting external stimuli and potential threats.

Hair Growth: Hair follicles on the scalp cycle through growth, rest, and shedding phases. This cyclical process, known as the hair growth cycle, ensures the continuous growth and replacement of hair.

Sebum Production: Sebaceous glands produce sebum, which moisturizes and protects the scalp and hair. However, overproduction or imbalance of sebum can contribute to conditions like dandruff or oily scalp.

Blood Supply: Rich vascularization in the scalp provides nutrients and oxygen to the hair follicles, supporting healthy hair growth.

In conclusion, the scalp's intricate anatomy and multi-faceted functions contribute significantly to overall health and well-being. Understanding its complexities helps in maintaining proper scalp care, ensuring healthy hair growth and overall comfort.

SKIN CELL TURNOVER

Skin cell turnover is a fundamental process that continuously renews and rejuvenates the skin. It involves the shedding of dead or damaged skin cells and the production of new ones, contributing to skin health, appearance, and protection.

Epidermis Layers: The epidermis, the outermost layer of the skin, comprises several sublayers, including the basal layer, spinous layer, granular layer, and stratum corneum. Cell turnover primarily occurs in the basal layer, where new skin cells, called keratinocytes, are formed.

Cell Renewal: Keratinocytes continuously divide and migrate upwards through the layers of the epidermis. As they move towards the surface, they undergo transformations, eventually becoming flattened, devoid of nuclei, and filled with a protein called keratin.

Shedding and Exfoliation: Once keratinocytes reach the stratum corneum, they form the outermost protective layer of the skin. These dead, flattened cells are shed through natural processes like washing, rubbing, or exfoliation.

Regulation of Turnover: Skin cell turnover is a tightly regulated process influenced by various factors such as age, hormones, genetics, and external factors like sun exposure or skincare products. Younger individuals generally have faster turnover rates, while aging can slow down this process.

Importance: Skin cell turnover is crucial for maintaining healthy, glowing skin. It helps in repairing damage, preventing clogged pores, reducing fine lines and wrinkles, and promoting an even skin tone.

Disruptions and Skin Conditions: Imbalances in cell turnover can lead to various skin conditions. For instance, increased turnover can cause conditions like psoriasis, where skin cells multiply too rapidly, leading to thickened, scaly patches. Conversely, reduced turnover can result in dull, rough skin or contribute to acne by clogging pores with dead cells.

In essence, skin cell turnover is a dynamic process vital for skin health and vitality. Understanding this process aids in choosing appropriate skincare routines and treatments to support and optimize skin renewal, promoting a healthier, more youthful appearance.

Chapter 3

TYPES OF DANDRUFF

THERE ARE MAINLY TWO TYPES OF DANDRUFF.

Dry dandruff: This type typically occurs when the scalp is dry, causing flaky skin to shed. It's often smaller in size and lighter in color.

Oily dandruff: This occurs when the scalp produces too much oil, leading to larger, greasy flakes. It's usually yellowish and sticks to the scalp and hair.

DRY SCALP VS. DANDRUFF

DRY SCALP:

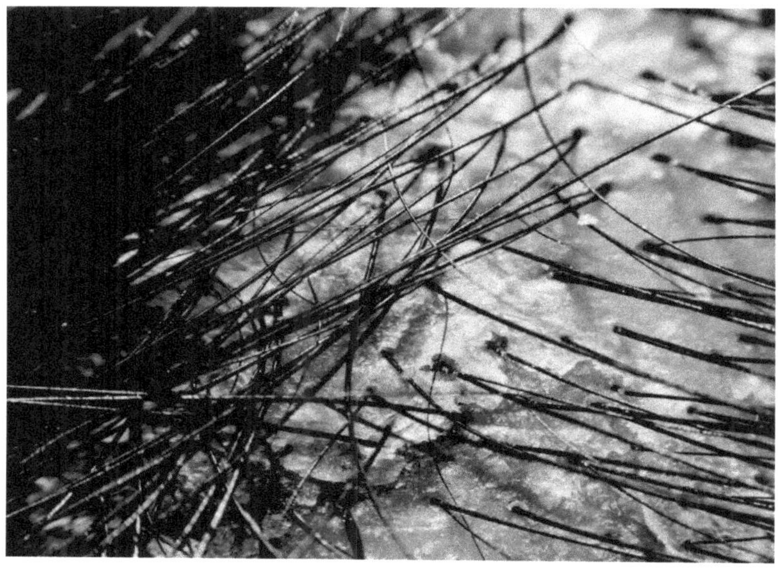

A dry scalp is often caused by environmental factors or insufficient moisture. It leads to the skin on the scalp becoming dry, resulting in itchiness and small, white flakes. Some common causes include cold weather, excessive shampooing, or using harsh hair products that strip the scalp of its natural oils. Symptoms may worsen with frequent exposure to heat, such as blow-drying.

DANDRUFF:

Dandruff, on the other hand, is a common scalp condition caused primarily by a fungus called Malassezia. It leads to the scalp shedding larger, oily or dry flakes that are more noticeable than those from a dry scalp. Dandruff can be influenced by factors such as stress, hormonal changes, improper hair hygiene, or a weakened immune system.

DISTINGUISHING FACTORS:

Flake Size and Texture: Dry scalp flakes are usually smaller and lighter, while dandruff flakes are larger, often oilier (in the case of oily dandruff), and may stick to the scalp and hair.

Scalp Condition: A dry scalp is generally just that—a lack of moisture affecting the scalp. Dandruff involves a more complex interaction of factors, including the presence of the fungus Malassezia, excess oil production, and irritation.

Causes: Dry scalp can be a result of external factors like weather or harsh hair products, while dandruff is often linked to a specific type of fungus, but other factors like stress or hormonal changes can also play a role.

TREATMENT:

For a dry scalp, using a gentle, moisturizing shampoo and conditioner can often alleviate symptoms. In contrast, dandruff might require specialized anti-dandruff shampoos containing ingredients like selenium sulfide, ketoconazole, zinc pyrithione, or salicylic acid to help manage the fungal overgrowth and reduce flakes.

It's essential to consult a trichologist or dermatologist or healthcare professional for a proper diagnosis and treatment plan tailored to the specific scalp condition.

Understanding the differences between a dry scalp and dandruff can help in choosing the right products and treatments to manage these conditions effectively.

OILY DANDRUFF OR SEBORRHEIC DERMATITIS

Seborrheic dermatitis is a common skin condition characterized by red, itchy, and flaky patches appearing on the skin. These patches can manifest on various areas of the body but commonly affect the scalp, face (particularly around the eyebrows, nose, and ears), and other oily regions like the chest and back.

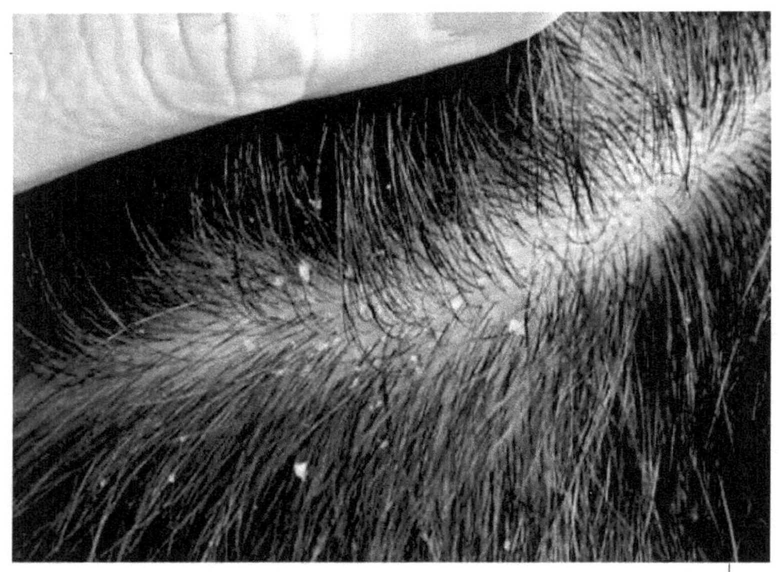

CAUSES AND TRIGGERS:

The precise cause of seborrheic dermatitis remains unclear, but factors such as overproduction of oil by the sebaceous glands, yeast (Malassezia) overgrowth on the skin, and individual genetic predispositions are believed to contribute to its development. Other factors like stress, hormones, neurological conditions, and certain illnesses can exacerbate the symptoms.

SYMPTOMS:

Seborrheic dermatitis often presents as red, inflamed skin covered with greasy or dry, white or yellow scales or flakes. The affected areas can itch intensely, leading to discomfort and sometimes a burning sensation. In infants, it's commonly referred to as "cradle cap," where yellowish, greasy scales appear on the scalp.

TREATMENT:

Treatment for seborrheic dermatitis typically involves a multifaceted approach. This can include medicated shampoos (containing ingredients like selenium sulfide, ketoconazole, zinc pyrithione), topical corticosteroids, antifungal creams, or medicated ointments to reduce inflammation and contro yeast growth. Gentle skincare routines and avoiding harsh products can also help manage symptoms.

MANAGING SEBORRHEIC DERMATITIS:

Since seborrheic dermatitis is often a chronic condition, managing it requires long-term strategies aimed at controlling flare-ups. This can involve regular use of prescribed treatments even when symptoms seem to subside, along with lifestyle adjustments to minimize triggers like stress, harsh weather conditions, or certain skincare products.

CONSULTING A PROFESSIONAL:

It's crucial to consult a trichologist or dermatologist or healthcare professional for an accurate diagnosis and tailored treatment plan. They can provide personalized guidance and suggest appropriate medications or lifestyle changes to effectively manage the condition.

In conclusion, while seborrheic dermatitis can be a persistent and sometimes uncomfortable skin condition, it is manageable with proper care, adherence to treatment regimens, and guidance from healthcare professionals. Understanding the triggers and symptoms can significantly aid in controlling the condition and improving the quality of life for those affected by it.

PSORIASIS AND DANDRUFF

PSORIASIS: UNDERSTANDING THE CONDITION

Psoriasis is a chronic autoimmune disorder characterized by the rapid buildup of skin cells, leading to the formation of thick, silvery scales and red patches. This condition occurs due to an accelerated skin cell growth cycle, causing cells to accumulate on the skin's surface. Psoriasis can affect any part of the body but commonly appears on the elbows, knees, scalp, and lower back.

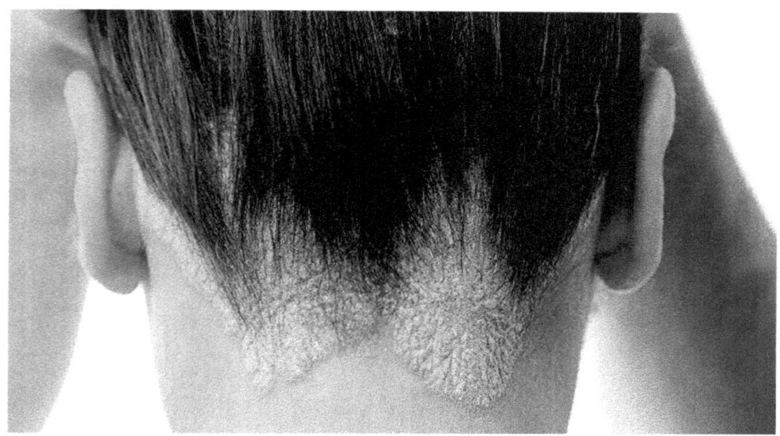

RELATIONSHIP BETWEEN PSORIASIS AND DANDRUFF:

While psoriasis and dandruff are distinct conditions, they both involve issues with the skin and can affect the scalp. Psoriasis of the scalp often appears as raised, red patches covered with silvery-white scales that extend beyond the hairline. This can sometimes be mistaken for severe dandruff due to the presence of flakes.

DIFFERENCES BETWEEN PSORIASIS AND DANDRUFF:

Underlying Cause: Psoriasis is an autoimmune condition, whereas dandruff is primarily caused by factors like a specific fungus (Malassezia), excess oil production, or dry scalp conditions.

Appearance: Psoriasis scales are usually thicker and silvery-white, covering a reddish base, while dandruff flakes tend to be smaller, white or yellowish, and can appear oily or dry.

Severity: Psoriasis often leads to thicker, more pronounced patches of scales and can be more persistent than dandruff.

TREATMENT:

While both conditions affect the scalp, the treatment approaches differ. Dandruff can often be managed with over-the-counter anti-dandruff shampoos containing active ingredients like zinc pyrithione, selenium sulfide, ketoconazole, or salicylic acid.

For scalp psoriasis, treatments may involve medicated shampoos containing coal tar, salicylic acid, or prescription-strength corticosteroids to reduce inflammation and slow down skin cell growth. In more severe cases, phototherapy or systemic medications prescribed by a dermatologist might be necessary.

Conclusion: Understanding the differences between psoriasis and dandruff is crucial for accurate diagnosis and appropriate treatment. While dandruff is a common scalp condition, psoriasis is a chronic autoimmune disorder requiring more targeted and specialized care. Consulting a healthcare professional or dermatologist for an accurate diagnosis and tailored treatment plan is essential for managing both conditions effectively and improving scalp health.

Chapter 4

SYMPTOMS AND DIAGNOSIS

Dandruff typically presents as white flakes in the hair and on the shoulders, caused by the shedding of dead skin cells from the scalp. Symptoms can include an itchy scalp and sometimes redness. Diagnosis is usually based on physical examination by a dermatologist or a healthcare professional that observes the scalp and considers the symptoms reported by the individual.

RECOGNIZING DANDRUFF

Recognizing dandruff is crucial for effective management and treatment. Dandruff manifests primarily through visible signs and physical sensations. Visually, it appears as white or yellowish flakes of dead skin on the scalp and hair. These flakes often fall onto clothing, causing embarrassment and discomfort.

Additionally, individuals with dandruff commonly experience an itchy scalp, which might lead to scratching. The scratching can aggravate the condition, causing redness and inflammation. In severe cases, the scalp might become dry and scaly, leading to further irritation.

Recognizing dandruff involves understanding these key indicators: the presence of flakes, itching, redness, and scalp discomfort. Identifying these signs promptly can prompt early intervention, leading to effective management strategies and alleviation of symptoms. Regular hair care, use of anti-dandruff shampoos, and maintaining a healthy scalp hygiene routine can significantly reduce dandruff's impact, promoting healthier and more comfortable scalp conditions.

MEDICAL EXAMINATIONS OF DANDRUFF

Medical examinations for dandruff are usually straightforward and often involve a physical examination of the scalp and hair by a healthcare professional. The diagnosis is primarily based on the appearance of the scalp and the characteristic flakes. In some cases, a dermatologist might use additional methods to confirm the diagnosis or rule out other conditions that may mimic dandruff symptoms.

During the examination, the healthcare provider inspects the scalp for the presence of white or yellowish flakes, redness, or signs of inflammation. They may use a tool like a Wood's lamp, which emits ultraviolet light, to assess the scalp more closely. This examination helps differentiate between dandruff and other conditions like scalp psoriasis or eczema, which might have similar symptoms.

In certain instances, if the diagnosis isn't evident or if the dandruff is unusually severe, the healthcare provider might perform a scalp biopsy. This involves taking a small sample of the scalp skin for further microscopic examination. However, this is not commonly required for typical dandruff cases.

It's essential for individuals experiencing persistent or severe dandruff to seek medical advice for accurate diagnosis and appropriate treatment. Medical examinations not only confirm the presence of dandruff but also help rule out other underlying scalp conditions, ensuring the right management strategy is employed to address the specific issue effectively.

DIFFERENTIAL DIAGNOSIS OF DANDRUFF

Differential diagnosis of dandruff involves distinguishing it from other conditions that exhibit similar symptoms. Several scalp conditions can present with flaking and itching, making it essential to differentiate dandruff from these potential alternatives.

Seborrheic Dermatitis: Often mistaken for dandruff due to similar flaking, seborrheic dermatitis involves more extensive inflammation and can affect areas beyond the scalp, such as the eyebrows, sides of the nose, and ears. It might require different treatment approaches than typical dandruff.

Scalp Psoriasis: Both psoriasis and dandruff can cause flaking, but psoriasis flakes are usually thicker, silver or whitish in color, and might be accompanied by red, inflamed patches. Scalp psoriasis tends to be more persistent and may extend beyond the hairline.

Fungal Infections: Conditions like tinea capitis, commonly known as scalp ringworm, can cause flaking similar to dandruff. However, ringworm typically results in patchy hair loss and might require antifungal treatment.

Allergic Reactions or Contact Dermatitis: Certain hair products or irritants can lead to an itchy, flaky scalp resembling dandruff. Identifying and avoiding these triggers can resolve the issue.

Eczema: Similar to seborrheic dermatitis, eczema can cause redness, itching, and flaking, often extending beyond the scalp area. It might require specific treatments based on its severity and cause.

Distinguishing dandruff from these conditions involves a comprehensive assessment of symptoms, their distribution, and sometimes additional diagnostic tests like skin biopsies or cultures. A healthcare professional's expertise is crucial in making an accurate diagnosis, as treatments can vary significantly based on the specific condition. Successful differentiation ensures appropriate and targeted management, relieving symptoms and promoting scalp health effectively.

Chapter 5

MANAGING DANDRUFF

Managing dandruff involves using anti-dandruff shampoos, maintaining good hygiene, avoiding stress, and following a balanced diet. Look for shampoos containing ingredients like zinc pyrithione, ketoconazole, or selenium sulfide, and consider regular scalp massages to improve blood circulation. If the issue persists, consult a dermatologist for personalized advice.

HOME REMEDIES AND OVER-THE-COUNTER TREATMENTS FOR DANDRUFF

Home remedies and over-the-counter treatments offer various options for managing dandruff effectively.

HOME REMEDIES:

Apple Cider Vinegar (ACV): Its acidity helps balance the pH of the scalp. Mix equal parts ACV and water, apply to the scalp, leave for 15-20 minutes, then rinse.

Tea Tree Oil: Known for its antifungal properties, mix a few drops with your shampoo or carrier oil and apply to the scalp.

Coconut Oil: Massaging warm coconut oil onto the scalp can moisturize and reduce flakiness.

Aloe Vera: Its antibacterial properties can soothe the scalp. Apply fresh aloe vera gel directly or use aloe-based shampoos.

Baking Soda: Gently exfoliates the scalp. Mix with water to form a paste, apply, and rinse thoroughly.

OVER-THE-COUNTER TREATMENTS:

Anti-dandruff Shampoos: Look for ingredients like zinc pyrithione, ketoconazole, selenium sulfide, coal tar, or salicylic acid. Use as directed on the label.

Coal Tar Shampoos: Effective against dandruff, but can discolor light-colored hair and have a strong odor.

Salicylic Acid Shampoos: Helps to eliminate scales and flakes.

Selenium Sulfide Shampoos: Slows down the growth of skin cells and reduces the yeast that contributes to dandruff.

Ketoconazole Shampoos: An antifungal agent that can effectively combat dandruff caused by fungi.

IMPORTANT NOTES:

Consistency: Both home remedies and over-the-counter treatments require consistent use for noticeable results.

Patch Test: Always do a patch test before trying any new product or home remedy to ensure you don't have adverse reactions.

MEDICAL TREATMENTS

Topical Steroid Solutions: For more severe cases, topical steroids may be prescribed to reduce inflammation and itching.

Coal Tar Preparations: Higher concentration coal tar solutions or treatments might be recommended for stubborn cases of dandruff or seborrheic dermatitis.

Laser Therapy: Some clinics offer laser treatments to reduce inflammation and promote a healthier scalp environment.

Nutritional Counseling: In some instances, nutritional deficiencies can contribute to dandruff. Nutritional counseling can help address these deficiencies through dietary changes or supplements.

IMPORTANT CONSIDERATIONS

Consultation: Always consult a dermatologist or healthcare professional before pursuing professional treatments or therapies for dandruff.

Personalized Approach: Professional treatments often involve a more targeted and personalized approach based on the severity and underlying cause of the dandruff.

Follow-up Care: Regular follow-ups and adherence to the treatment plan are crucial to achieving and maintaining results.

Medical treatments and therapies for dandruff offer more advanced and targeted approaches for individuals struggling with persistent or severe dandruff, providing specialized solutions tailored to their specific needs and conditions.

LIFESTYLE CHANGES FOR PREVENTION OF DANDRUFF

Making certain lifestyle changes can significantly contribute to preventing dandruff and maintaining a healthy scalp.

1. HYGIENE PRACTICES:

Regular Hair Washing: Frequent washing with a mild shampoo helps remove excess oil and dead skin cells, preventing buildup.
Proper Rinsing: Ensure thorough rinsing to remove all traces of shampoo and conditioner, which can otherwise contribute to scalp irritation.

2. DIET AND NUTRITION:

Balanced Diet: A diet rich in nutrients, especially zinc, B vitamins, and omega-3 fatty acids, promotes a healthy scalp.

Hydration: Drinking an adequate amount of water helps maintain scalp moisture and overall skin health.

3. STRESS MANAGEMENT:

Stress Reduction: Stress can exacerbate dandruff. Techniques like meditation, yoga, or regular exercise can help manage stress levels.

4. HAIR CARE PRACTICES:

Avoiding Heat and Chemicals: Excessive use of styling tools, hair dyes, and harsh chemicals can irritate the scalp and contribute to dandruff.

Using Gentle Products: Opt for mild, gentle shampoos and conditioners that suit your scalp type.

5. SCALP CARE ROUTINE:

Regular Scalp Massage: Promotes blood circulation and helps prevent the buildup of dead skin cells.

Exfoliation: Gentle exfoliation using natural methods like brushing or exfoliating masks can reduce flakes and prevent buildup.

6. AVOIDING TRIGGERS:

Identify Allergens or Irritants: Some individuals might have specific triggers like certain foods or allergens that exacerbate dandruff. Identifying and avoiding these can be helpful.

7. REGULAR CHECK-UPS:

Dermatologist Consultation: Regular visits to a dermatologist can help identify any underlying scalp conditions early on and prevent them from worsening.

By adopting these lifestyle changes, individuals can proactively manage and prevent dandruff, maintaining a healthier scalp and reducing the likelihood of persistent flaking and itching.

SPECIAL CASES AND CONSIDERATIONS

DANDRUFF IN CHILDREN

Dandruff, a common scalp condition characterized by flaky skin, affects not only adults but also children. While it may not pose significant health risks, it can cause discomfort and self-consciousness in children. Understanding the causes, symptoms, and effective management of dandruff in this age group is crucial for their well-being.

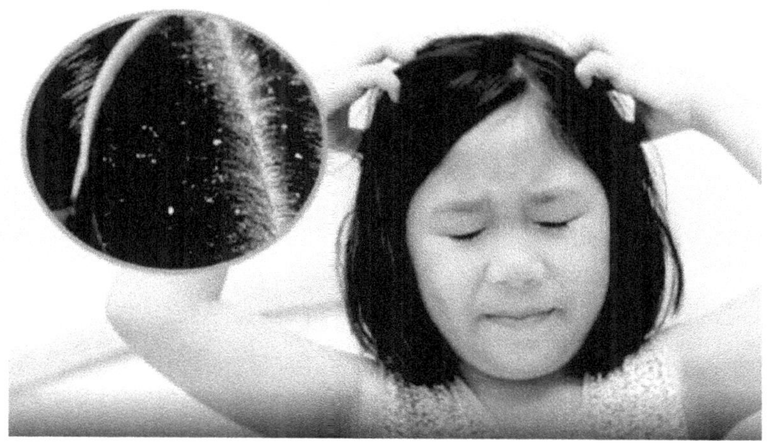

CAUSES AND SYMPTOMS

Dandruff in children can stem from various factors. One primary cause is the overgrowth of a naturally occurring fungus called Malassezia on the scalp. This overgrowth leads to irritation and accelerated shedding of skin cells, resulting in the characteristic white or yellowish flakes on the scalp and hair.

Other factors such as sensitivity to certain hair products, infrequent washing, or underlying skin conditions like eczema or psoriasis can contribute to dandruff in children.

SYMPTOMS OF DANDRUFF IN CHILDREN OFTEN MANIFEST AS:

- ✓ WHITE OR YELLOW FLAKES ON THE SCALP OR HAIR
- ✓ ITCHY AND IRRITATED SCALP
- ✓ DRYNESS OR OILINESS ON THE SCALP
- ✓ REDNESS OR INFLAMMATION IN SEVERE CASES
- ✓ MANAGEMENT AND TREATMENT

Managing dandruff in children primarily involves maintaining proper scalp hygiene and using appropriate hair care products. Regular, gentle washing of the hair with mild, anti-dandruff shampoos suitable for children is essential. These shampoos often contain ingredients like pyrithione zinc, selenium sulfide, or ketoconazole to combat the fungus causing dandruff.

However, it's crucial to use these products as directed and avoid excessive washing, which can strip the scalp of its natural oils, potentially worsening the condition.

Apart from hygiene, dietary adjustments and managing stress levels might also contribute to reducing dandruff. A balanced diet rich in vitamins and minerals can promote a healthy scalp.

In cases where dandruff persists despite home care, consulting a pediatrician or a dermatologist is advisable. They can assess the severity of the condition and recommend suitable treatment, which might include medicated shampoos or topical treatments tailored for children.

Conclusion: While dandruff in children might not be a severe medical issue, it can affect their self-esteem and comfort. By understanding the causes and symptoms and adopting appropriate management strategies, parents can help their children effectively deal with dandruff. Regular scalp care, suitable hair products, and, if necessary, professional guidance can ensure that children can enjoy a healthy scalp and hair without the discomfort and embarrassment associated with dandruff.

THE PSYCHOLOGICAL IMPACT OF DANDRUFF

Dandruff, a seemingly innocuous scalp condition characterized by flaking skin, often extends beyond its physical manifestations, significantly impacting an individual's psychological well-being. Though not a serious medical concern, the social stigma, embarrassment, and psychological effects associated with dandruff can affect one's self-esteem and overall quality of life.

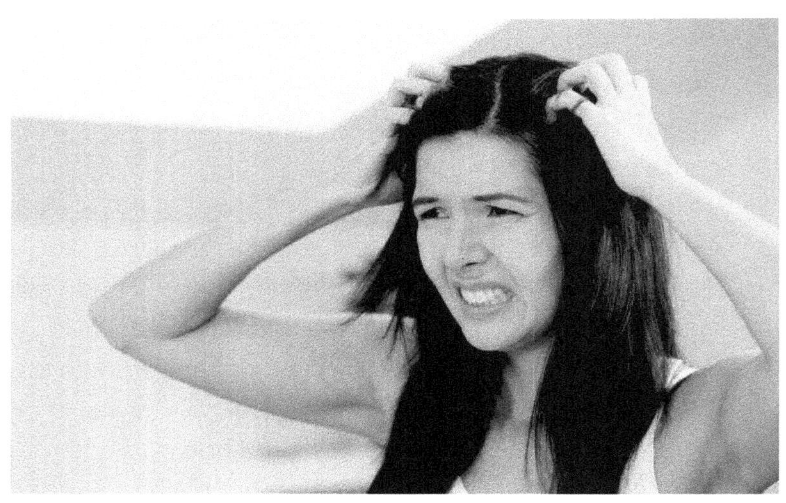

SOCIAL STIGMA AND SELF-IMAGE

The visible flakes on clothing, shoulders, and hair draw unwanted attention, leading to social discomfort and self-consciousness. Individuals with dandruff may experience embarrassment or a sense of uncleanliness, adversely affecting their confidence and social interactions. Persistent worries about others noticing the flakes or perceiving them negatively can lead to withdrawal from social situations, impacting relationships and personal development, particularly in adolescents.

SELF-ESTEEM AND CONFIDENCE

The perception of dandruff as a hygiene issue or lack of proper care often affects self-esteem. Constant concerns about one's appearance, fear of judgment, or feelings of inadequacy can significantly erode self-confidence. This diminished self-assurance might extend beyond the visible symptoms, affecting various aspects of life, such as academic performance, career opportunities, or forming new relationships.

PSYCHOLOGICAL DISTRESS

The chronic nature of dandruff, despite attempts to manage it, can induce stress, anxiety, or even depression in some individuals. The persistent cycle of treating and experiencing recurring flakes can lead to frustration and feelings of helplessness. This emotional burden might further exacerbate the condition due to the potential correlation between stress and increased dandruff severity.

MANAGEMENT AND COPING STRATEGIES

Effective management of dandruff not only involves addressing the physical symptoms but also mitigating its psychological impact. Encouraging open communication about dandruff, normalizing its prevalence, and providing education about its causes and treatments can alleviate the stigma associated with it.

Moreover, adopting coping strategies such as stress management techniques, seeking support from friends, family, or mental health professionals, and focusing on one's overall well-being can help individuals navigate the psychological challenges associated with dandruff.

Conclusion: While dandruff might seem like a minor dermatological issue, its psychological ramifications can significantly affect an individual's mental health and quality of life. Empathy, understanding, and efforts to destigmatize dandruff play a crucial role in supporting affected individuals. Recognizing the psychological toll and addressing both the physical symptoms and emotional impact can aid in restoring confidence and improving the overall mental well-being of those grappling with dandruff.

Chapter 7

FUTURE PERSPECTIVES

In recent years, ongoing research has focused on developing more effective treatments for dandruff, including understanding its root causes better. Advances in understanding scalp health, microbiome studies, and technology might bring about improved and personalized treatments, possibly using probiotics, targeted therapies, or innovative products. There's also a growing emphasis on sustainable and natural remedies for scalp conditions, which might influence future dandruff solutions.

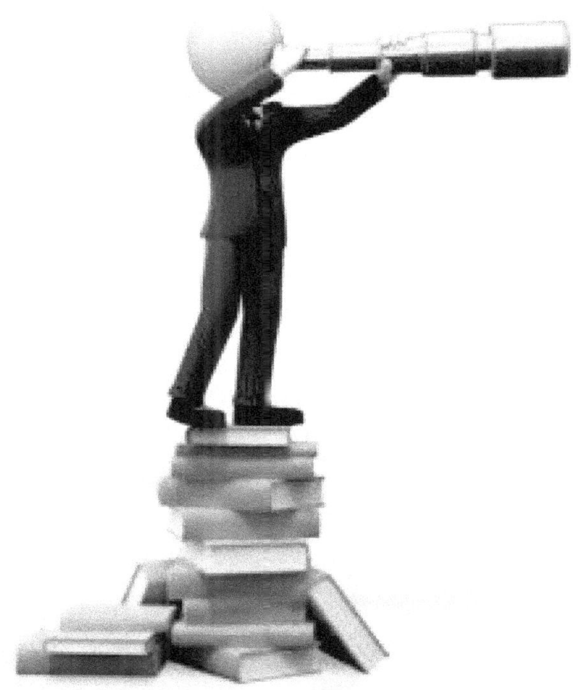

ONGOING RESEARCH ON DANDRUFF

Dandruff, a prevalent scalp condition affecting millions worldwide, continues to be a subject of extensive research and study. In recent years, the scientific community has made significant strides in unraveling the complexities surrounding dandruff, focusing on its etiology, microbial involvement, and novel treatment approaches.

One of the fundamental areas of ongoing research revolves around comprehending the underlying causes of dandruff. Historically perceived as simply a result of dry scalp, modern studies have shifted focus towards the intricate interplay between host factors, scalp microbiota, and environmental influences. Researchers have identified specific fungi, particularly Malassezia species, as key contributors to dandruff. Understanding the interaction between these microbes and the scalp's immune response has become pivotal in developing targeted treatments.

Microbiome studies have emerged as a crucial aspect of dandruff research. The scalp's microbiome, akin to the gut microbiome's significance to overall health, is being extensively explored. Scientists are delving into the diversity and dynamics of microbial populations on the scalp, seeking correlations between certain microbial imbalances and dandruff severity. This avenue of research holds promise for tailored interventions aiming to restore a healthy scalp microbiome, potentially revolutionizing dandruff management.

Furthermore, ongoing advancements in technology are reshaping the approach to dandruff treatment. Innovations in molecular biology, such as genomic sequencing and metagenomic analyses, allow for a deeper understanding of the genetic makeup of Malassezia and other scalp microorganisms. This knowledge aids in the development of targeted therapies that specifically address the mechanisms driving dandruff formation.

In parallel, the quest for more effective and safer treatments has led researchers to explore alternative solutions. Natural remedies and botanical extracts are gaining attention for their potential anti-dandruff properties. Substances like tea tree oil, aloe vera, and certain plant-based compounds show promising results in mitigating dandruff symptoms without the side effects associated with conventional treatments.

Moreover, the growing emphasis on sustainability and eco-friendliness in skincare products has influenced ongoing research in dandruff treatments. Scientists are investigating eco-conscious formulations that not only effectively combat dandruff but also minimize environmental impact, catering to a more environmentally aware consumer base.

In conclusion, the ongoing research on dandruff is multifaceted and dynamic, encompassing various scientific disciplines. As our understanding of the scalp microbiome, microbial interactions, and treatment technologies continues to evolve, it holds the promise of delivering more targeted, efficient, and sustainable solutions for managing dandruff, potentially offering relief to individuals plagued by this common scalp condition.

POTENTIAL BREAKTHROUGHS IN DANDRUFF TREATMENT

Dandruff, a common scalp condition, has long been a source of frustration for many individuals worldwide. However, the landscape of dandruff treatment is on the brink of significant breakthroughs, fueled by ongoing research and advancements in various scientific domains.

One of the most promising areas of breakthrough lies in the deeper understanding of the scalp microbiome and its relationship with dandruff. Recent studies have elucidated the complex interplay between scalp microorganisms, particularly Malassezia species, and the host immune response. This understanding has opened avenues for developing targeted therapies that aim to modulate the scalp microbiome, potentially providing long-lasting relief from dandruff.

Probiotic and prebiotic formulations tailored to restore a healthy scalp microbiota represent a potential breakthrough in dandruff treatment. These formulations, designed to promote the growth of beneficial microorganisms while suppressing dandruff-causing fungi, offer a more holistic and sustainable approach compared to conventional treatments.

Moreover, advancements in technology, particularly in genomic sequencing and metagenomic analyses, have paved the way for personalized dandruff treatments. The ability to analyze an individual's scalp microbiota, genetic predispositions, and specific microbial imbalances could revolutionize treatment strategies. Personalized medicine approaches could lead to highly targeted therapies, optimizing treatment efficacy while minimizing adverse effects.

Another exciting avenue involves the exploration of novel active ingredients derived from natural sources. Compounds like plant extracts, essential oils, and herbal formulations with potent antimicrobial and anti-inflammatory properties show promise in managing dandruff effectively. These natural remedies not only address dandruff symptoms but also offer a gentle and sustainable alternative to traditional treatments.

Furthermore, the convergence of nanotechnology and skincare presents an intriguing possibility for breakthroughs in dandruff treatment. Nano-based delivery systems allow for enhanced penetration of active ingredients into the scalp, potentially improving treatment efficacy and providing longer-lasting relief.

Additionally, the development of innovative and sustainable formulations aligns with the growing demand for eco-friendly skincare products. Researchers are exploring eco-conscious solutions that combat dandruff while minimizing environmental impact, catering to a more environmentally conscious consumer base.

In conclusion, the pursuit of breakthroughs in dandruff treatment encompasses diverse fronts, from microbiome research to personalized medicine and sustainable innovations. The potential breakthroughs in manipulating the scalp microbiome, personalized therapies, natural remedies, nanotechnology-driven treatments, and eco-friendly formulations hold promise for transforming the landscape of dandruff management. These breakthroughs could herald a new era of highly effective, personalized, and sustainable solutions, offering hope to individuals seeking lasting relief from the challenges posed by dandruff.

FAQS ABOUT DANDRUFF

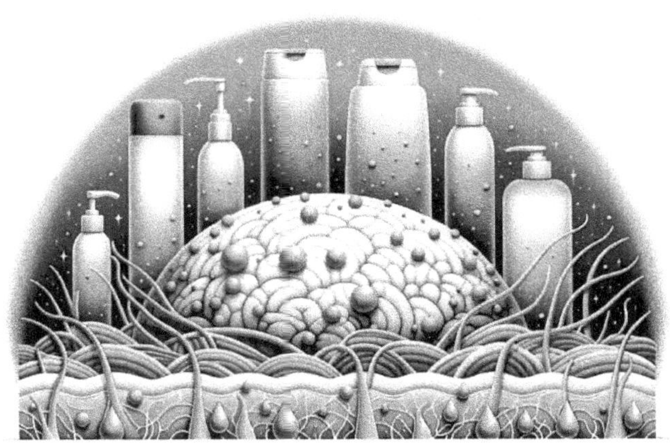

WHAT IS DANDRUFF?

Dandruff is a common scalp condition characterized by the flaking of dead skin cells from the scalp. It can lead to an itchy scalp and visible white or yellowish flakes on the hair and shoulders.

WHAT CAUSES DANDRUFF?

Dandruff can be caused by various factors such as an overgrowth of yeast-like fungus, dry skin, sensitivity to hair products, certain skin conditions like eczema or psoriasis, hormonal changes, stress, or a lack of proper hair hygiene.

IS DANDRUFF CONTAGIOUS?

No, dandruff is not contagious. It's a scalp condition and cannot be passed from person to person.

CAN DANDRUFF LEAD TO HAIR LOSS?

Dandruff itself doesn't typically cause hair loss. However, persistent scratching of the scalp due to itching caused by dandruff can potentially damage hair follicles and lead to hair breakage.

HOW IS DANDRUFF TREATED?

Treatment options for dandruff include using medicated anti-dandruff shampoos containing active ingredients like selenium sulfide, zinc pyrithione, ketoconazole, coal tar, or salicylic acid. Maintaining good scalp hygiene, managing stress, and avoiding harsh hair products can also help.

HOW OFTEN SHOULD I WASH MY HAIR TO CONTROL DANDRUFF?

Washing your hair regularly, at least two to three times a week, with an anti-dandruff shampoo can help control dandruff. However, individual needs may vary, and it's essential to find a balance that works for your scalp.

CAN CERTAIN FOODS CAUSE DANDRUFF?

There's no direct link between specific foods and dandruff. However, some people believe that certain foods high in sugar, unhealthy fats, or processed foods might exacerbate dandruff symptoms.

ARE THERE NATURAL REMEDIES FOR DANDRUFF?

Some natural remedies that may help reduce dandruff include tea tree oil, coconut oil, aloe vera, apple cider vinegar rinses, and maintaining a balanced diet with adequate hydration.

CAN DANDRUFF AFFECT OTHER PARTS OF THE BODY?
Dandruff primarily affects the scalp, but in some cases, it can also occur in other oily areas with skin, such as the eyebrows, sides of the nose, ears, chest, and back.

WHEN SHOULD I SEE A DOCTOR FOR DANDRUFF?

If over-the-counter shampoos and home remedies don't improve your dandruff or if it worsens, consult a dermatologist or a healthcare professional for a proper diagnosis and treatment plan.

IS DANDRUFF ONLY A WINTER PROBLEM?

While dandruff can sometimes worsen in dry, cold weather due to the scalp becoming dry, it's not solely a winter problem. Dandruff can occur at any time of the year due to various causes.

CAN STRESS CAUSE DANDRUFF?

Stress can contribute to dandruff or exacerbate existing dandruff symptoms. It can weaken the immune system, making the scalp more susceptible to various conditions that lead to dandruff.

CAN DANDRUFF BE PREVENTED?

While it may not always be possible to prevent dandruff entirely, maintaining good scalp hygiene, using gentle shampoos, managing stress levels, eating a balanced diet, and avoiding triggers that worsen dandruff can help minimize its occurrence.

CAN I USE REGULAR SHAMPOO TO TREAT DANDRUFF?

Regular shampoos may not effectively treat dandruff as they might not have specific active ingredients targeting the underlying causes. Anti-dandruff shampoos are formulated with active ingredients to address dandruff more effectively.

CAN DANDRUFF AFFECT CHILDREN?

Yes, dandruff can affect children as well. It's known as pediatric seborrheic dermatitis, characterized by similar symptoms to adult dandruff, such as flaky scalp and itching.

CAN CHANGING HAIR CARE PRODUCTS HELP WITH DANDRUFF?

Switching to hair care products that are gentle and formulated for sensitive scalps or specifically designed to combat dandruff might help alleviate symptoms. However, it's essential to find products that work well for your scalp and hair type.

IS THERE A LINK BETWEEN DANDRUFF AND OILY HAIR?

There can be a link between dandruff and oily hair. Some individuals with oily scalps might be more prone to dandruff because the excess oil can contribute to the growth of Malassezia, a yeast-like fungus associated with dandruff.

CAN DANDRUFF CAUSE SCALP INFECTIONS?

If left untreated for a prolonged period, severe dandruff or certain underlying conditions causing dandruff can potentially lead to secondary scalp infections. It's crucial to address dandruff to prevent such complications.

CAN DANDRUFF AFFECT PEOPLE OF ALL AGES?

Yes, dandruff can affect people of all ages, from infants to the elderly. It's a common scalp condition that can occur at any stage of life.

CAN HORMONAL CHANGES CAUSE DANDRUFF?

Hormonal changes, especially during puberty or due to conditions like hormonal imbalances or pregnancy, can sometimes trigger or worsen dandruff.

CAN EXCESSIVE WASHING CAUSE DANDRUFF?

Excessive washing, especially with harsh shampoos that strip the scalp of natural oils, can lead to dryness and potentially exacerbate dandruff. Finding a balance in washing frequency and using mild shampoos is essential.

Can dandruff be a symptom of a more serious health condition?

In most cases, dandruff is a benign scalp condition. However, in rare instances, it can be a symptom of an underlying health condition such as seborrheic dermatitis, psoriasis, or fungal infections. Consulting a doctor can help rule out any serious underlying issues.

CAN DYEING OR COLORING HAIR WORSEN DANDRUFF?

Chemical treatments like hair dyeing or coloring may irritate the scalp and potentially worsen dandruff symptoms in some individuals. Opting for gentle or natural hair coloring methods might be preferable for those prone to dandruff.

HOW LONG DOES IT TAKE TO GET RID OF DANDRUFF?

The time it takes to get rid of dandruff varies from person to person. With proper treatment and consistent use of anti-dandruff products, some individuals may see improvements in a few weeks, while others might take longer.

CAN EXCESSIVE SWEATING WORSEN DANDRUFF?

Excessive sweating can sometimes contribute to dandruff, as the sweat can mix with natural oils and lead to scalp irritation. However, regular washing and maintaining good hygiene can help mitigate this effect.

CAN DANDRUFF CAUSE AN ALLERGIC REACTION?

Dandruff itself is not an allergic reaction. However, some people might have sensitivities or allergies to certain ingredients in anti-dandruff shampoos, leading to scalp irritation or allergic reactions.

CAN DANDRUFF BE HEREDITARY?

There might be a genetic predisposition to dandruff. If one or both parents have had dandruff, their children might be more likely to develop it as well.

CAN SWIMMING IN CHLORINATED POOLS WORSEN DANDRUFF?

Chlorinated pools can sometimes dry out the scalp, potentially exacerbating dandruff in some individuals. Rinsing hair thoroughly after swimming and using a moisturizing shampoo can help mitigate this effect.

CAN DANDRUFF CAUSE PSYCHOLOGICAL EFFECTS?

For some individuals, persistent dandruff can lead to self-consciousness or embarrassment, affecting their self-esteem and confidence levels. Seeking effective treatment and support can help manage these psychological effects.

CAN DANDRUFF BE PRESENT WITHOUT VISIBLE FLAKES?

Yes, dandruff can exist without noticeable flakes. Sometimes, it's more about scalp irritation, itchiness, or redness without the typical visible flaking.

CAN USING TOO MANY HAIR STYLING PRODUCTS CAUSE DANDRUFF?

Certain hair styling products containing harsh chemicals or excessive build-up might contribute to scalp irritation, leading to dandruff-like symptoms. Using these products in moderation and ensuring proper cleansing might help prevent this.

CAN ALLERGIES CONTRIBUTE TO DANDRUFF?

Allergies, especially to certain hair care products or ingredients within them, might cause scalp irritation resembling dandruff. Identifying and avoiding these allergens can alleviate symptoms.

CAN PETS CAUSE DANDRUFF IN HUMANS?

Pets can carry dander, dead skin flakes, which may cause allergic reactions in some people. However, human dandruff and pet dander are not directly related.

CAN DANDRUFF DEVELOP SUDDENLY?

While dandruff often develops gradually, certain factors like hormonal changes, stress, or shifts in weather conditions might trigger sudden or acute instances of dandruff.

CAN DANDRUFF CAUSE PIMPLES OR ACNE ON THE SCALP?

In some cases, severe dandruff or conditions related to it, like seborrheic dermatitis, might lead to scalp pimples or acne-like eruptions. Proper treatment can help alleviate these symptoms.

CAN FREQUENT SCRATCHING WORSEN DANDRUFF?

Frequent scratching of the scalp due to dandruff-related itchiness can cause inflammation and potentially worsen dandruff. It's important to avoid excessive scratching to prevent irritation.

CAN DANDRUFF AFFECT HAIR TEXTURE?

Chronic or severe dandruff might cause some damage to hair strands, leading to brittleness or changes in texture. However, this is usually a result of persistent scratching or underlying scalp conditions.

CAN NATURAL HAIR CONTRIBUTE TO DANDRUFF?

Natural hair, especially coarser textures, might be prone to dandruff due to the hair's structure and potential difficulty in distributing natural oils evenly along the scalp.

CAN HORMONAL CHANGES DURING MENOPAUSE WORSEN DANDRUFF?

Fluctuating hormones during menopause can affect the skin, potentially leading to changes in the scalp's oil production, which might exacerbate dandruff in some women.